TABLE OF CONTENT

DISCLAIMER

The information provided in this book is for general informational purposes only. While the author has made every effort to ensure the accuracy and completeness of the content, they do not warrant or represent its accuracy. The author and the publisher assume no responsibility for errors or omissions or for any consequences resulting from the use of the information contained herein. Readers are advised to consult with appropriate professionals for specific advice tailored to their situation. The views and opinions expressed in this book are those of the author and do not necessarily reflect the official policy or position of any organization or entity mentioned. The author and the publisher disclaim any liability, loss, or risk incurred as a consequence, directly or indirectly, of the use and application of any of the contents of this book.

COPYRIGHT

EMBRACING THE CHILL

A GUIDE TO THRIVING IN WINTER'S GRASPS

MERCY GRACE

INTRODUCTION

Winter, with its crisp air and glistening snow, paints a serene picture of a seasonal wonderland. However, as the temperature drops and frost blankets the world, the cold season brings its own set of challenges to our physical and mental well-being. Staying healthy and thriving in the cold requires a holistic approach that considers the unique aspects of winter living. In this comprehensive guide, we'll explore strategies and practices to not only weather the winter but to embrace it with vitality and resilience.

The winter months often coincide with festivities, holidays, and a sense of coziness. Yet, beneath the enchanting facade lies the potential for seasonal ailments, reduced physical activity, and a shift in mood. Winter wellness is about acknowledging these challenges and proactively adopting habits that nourish both body and mind.

As the days grow shorter and the nights longer, maintaining a balance becomes essential. From bolstering your immune system to embracing physical activities suited for the season, and from nurturing your skin against the cold winds to cultivating mental resilience, this guide is a roadmap to navigating the winter months with intentionality.

Winter is not just a season; it's an opportunity for introspection, self-care, and the cultivation of habits that will carry you through the cold and into the blossoming warmth of spring. Join us on this journey to discover the art of thriving in the cold, finding joy in winter's unique offerings, and emerging on the other side with a renewed sense of well-being. Let's dive into the strategies that will make this winter a season of not just survival but of thriving in the face of the frosty embrace.

Winter invites us to pause, reflect, and adapt our lifestyles to align with the rhythm of the season. It's a time to cocoon ourselves in self-care practices that not only shield us from the harshness of winter but also allow us to emerge stronger, healthier, and more connected to the beauty that lies within the frosty landscape.

Throughout this guide, we'll explore the multifaceted aspects of winter wellness, touching on the physical, mental, and emotional elements that collectively contribute to a holistic state of well-being. From fortifying your immune system against seasonal illnesses to discovering the joy of winter-friendly physical activities, each chapter is designed to equip you with practical strategies to thrive in the cold.

Winter is not a season to merely endure; it's an opportunity to embrace the unique gifts it brings. The chill in the air invites us to savor warming soups, engage in invigorating outdoor activities, and foster connections with loved ones around cozy fires. As we navigate the challenges of winter living, we'll uncover the hidden treasures that lie beneath the frost and snow.

The journey to winter wellness is a personal one, shaped by individual preferences, experiences, and aspirations. Whether you find solace in the stillness of a snowy landscape, the warmth of a mug filled with herbal tea, or the joy of shared laughter on a cold night, this guide is designed to inspire you to create your own narrative of thriving in the cold.

So, as winter unfolds its icy embrace, let's embark on a transformative journey together. Embrace the beauty of the season, nurture your body and mind, and discover the resilience that comes from aligning with the ebb and flow of winter. Let the frost be not a barrier but a canvas upon which you paint a tapestry of well-being, turning the cold into an opportunity for growth, connection, and thriving in the midst of winter's enchantment.

CHAPTER ONE : BOOSTING IMMUNITY:

As winter settles in, bolstering your immune system becomes paramount in staying healthy and

resilient against seasonal illnesses. The cold weather and decreased sunlight can pose

challenges to our well-being, making it essential to adopt immune-boosting practices. In this

guide, we delve deeper into effective strategies for fortifying your immune system during the

winter months.

- NUTRIENT-RICH FOODS:

Incorporate a variety of fruits and vegetables into your diet, focusing on those rich in vitamins C

and E, as well as zinc.

Include citrus fruits, berries, spinach, broccoli, almonds, and seeds in your meals.

Explore immune-boosting herbs and spices such as ginger, garlic, and turmeric.

Hydration with Warm Beverages:

Stay hydrated by drinking plenty of water throughout the day.

Include warm beverages like herbal teas, broths, and warm water with lemon to support

hydration and soothe the respiratory system.

Limit the consumption of dehydrating substances such as excessive caffeine and alcohol.

- PROBIOTICS AND GUT HEALTH:

Consume probiotic-rich foods like yogurt, kefir, sauerkraut, and kimchi to promote a healthy gut

microbiome.

Consider taking probiotic supplements to enhance gut flora, which plays a crucial role in

immune function.

Ensure a diet high in fiber to support digestive health.

- ADEQUATE VITAMIN D INTAKE:

Since sunlight exposure may be limited during winter, consider vitamin D supplements or

include vitamin D-rich foods like fatty fish, fortified dairy products, and egg yolks in your diet.

A balanced vitamin D level contributes to a robust immune response.

- **REGULAR EXERCISE:**

Engage in moderate-intensity exercise, such as walking, jogging, or indoor workouts, to promote

circulation and overall health.

Regular physical activity has been shown to enhance immune function and reduce the risk of

infections.

- **ADEQUATE SLEEP:**

Prioritize quality sleep by maintaining a consistent sleep schedule.

Create a sleep-conducive environment, including a dark and quiet room, to support restful

sleep.

Lack of sleep can compromise immune function, so aim for 7-9 hours of sleep per night.

- **STRESS MANAGEMENT:**

Practice stress-reducing techniques such as meditation, deep breathing exercises, or yoga.

Chronic stress can weaken the immune system, so incorporating relaxation practices is crucial

for winter wellness.

- STAY HYGIENIC:

Practice good hygiene, including regular handwashing, to reduce the risk of infections.

Keep your surroundings clean and disinfect frequently-touched surfaces.

Avoid close contact with sick individuals and practice respiratory hygiene.

Prioritizing immune health is a proactive and effective approach to staying healthy during the

winter months. By adopting a balanced lifestyle that includes nutrient-dense foods, hydration,

regular exercise, and stress management, you can strengthen your immune system and

navigate the winter season with resilience and vitality. Embrace these immune-boosting

practices to fortify your body against seasonal challenges and enjoy a healthy winter.

CHAPTER TWO : MAINTAINING PHYSICAL ACTIVITY:

Staying active during the winter months is not only essential for maintaining physical health but

also for uplifting your mood and combating the winter blues. The colder weather may present

challenges, but with a bit of creativity and motivation, you can embrace a variety of

winter-friendly exercises to keep your body in motion. In this guide, we explore effective

strategies for maintaining physical activity during the winter season.

- WINTER-FRIENDLY OUTDOOR ACTIVITIES:

Engage in winter sports such as skiing, snowboarding, ice skating, or snowshoeing.

Take advantage of snowy landscapes for activities like building snowmen, having snowball

fights, or going on winter hikes.

Consider joining a local winter sports club or group for added motivation and social interaction.

- **INDOOR WORKOUT ROUTINES:**

Create a home workout space with minimal equipment, incorporating exercises like squats,

lunges, push-ups, and planks.

Explore online workout classes or fitness apps that offer guided workouts suitable for indoor

spaces.

Invest in indoor exercise equipment such as a stationary bike, treadmill, or resistance bands for

a diverse workout routine.

- **FLEXIBILITY AND MOBILITY EXERCISES:**

Incorporate flexibility exercises to maintain joint health and prevent stiffness.

Practice yoga or Pilates, both of which offer a combination of flexibility, strength, and relaxation.

Dedicate a few minutes each day to stretching exercises to improve overall flexibility.

- **DANCE AND AEROBIC WORKOUTS:**

Join a dance class or engage in dance workouts at home to add a fun and energetic element to your routine.

Participate in aerobic exercises to elevate your heart rate and boost cardiovascular health.

Create themed playlists to make your workouts more enjoyable and dynamic.

- WINTER SPORTS LEAGUES AND CLASSES:

Explore local sports leagues or classes specifically designed for the winter season.

Join a winter swimming club or water aerobics class for a refreshing and invigorating workout.

Enroll in indoor sports such as basketball, volleyball, or racquet sports to stay active and

socialize.

- FITNESS CHALLENGES AND GOALS:

Set achievable fitness goals for the winter season, whether it's increasing daily step counts,

improving endurance, or mastering a new exercise.

Join virtual fitness challenges or competitions to stay motivated and connected with a

community.

Track your progress using fitness apps or a journal to celebrate achievements and stay

accountable.

- WINTER GARDENING AND OUTDOOR CHORES:

Embrace winter gardening activities, such as pruning, planting winter crops, or maintaining

outdoor spaces.

Engage in outdoor chores like shoveling snow, which provides a full-body workout.

Incorporate functional movements into everyday tasks to promote physical activity.

- STAY ACTIVE WITH FAMILY AND FRIENDS:

Organize group activities with family or friends, such as a friendly game of winter sports or a

nature walk.

Schedule regular workout sessions with a workout buddy to enhance motivation and

accountability.

Plan active social gatherings to combine physical activity with quality time spent with loved

ones.

Maintaining physical activity during the winter season is not only achievable but can also be

enjoyable and invigorating. Whether you prefer indoor workouts, outdoor adventures, or a mix of

both, finding activities that suit your preferences will help you stay active and healthy throughout

the colder months. Embrace the winter landscape as an opportunity to explore new activities,

set fitness goals, and prioritize your overall well-being.

CHAPTER THREE :
COLD-WEATHER SKIN CARE:

The winter season brings not only a picturesque snowy landscape but also colder temperatures

that can take a toll on your skin. Harsh winds, low humidity, and indoor heating can lead to

dryness, irritation, and other skin concerns. In this guide, we'll explore effective strategies for

maintaining healthy and radiant skin during the winter months.

- HYDRATING SKIN MOISTURIZERS:

Invest in a rich and hydrating moisturizer to combat dryness caused by the cold weather.

Opt for moisturizers containing ingredients like hyaluronic acid, glycerin, or shea butter for deep

hydration.

Apply moisturizer immediately after bathing to lock in moisture and prevent skin dehydration.

Gentle Cleansing Routine:

Use a mild and hydrating cleanser to cleanse your face and body without stripping away natural

oils.
Limit hot showers, as hot water can contribute to skin
dryness. Opt for lukewarm water instead.

Pat your skin dry gently with a soft towel after cleansing to
avoid irritation.

- PROTECTIVE CLOTHING:

Wear protective clothing, such as scarves, gloves, and
hats, to shield your skin from the cold

winds.

Choose fabrics like cotton and wool for winter clothing, as
they provide warmth without causing

excessive irritation.

Don't forget sunscreen, even in winter, to protect your skin
from UV rays that can still be

harmful, especially in snowy conditions.

- HUMIDIFIER USE:

Incorporate a humidifier into your indoor environment to
combat the dry air caused by heating

systems.

Maintain optimal indoor humidity levels to prevent skin dryness and irritation.
Place humidifiers in commonly used areas, such as bedrooms and living rooms, for maximum

effectiveness.

- EXFOLIATION WITH CAUTION:

Limit exfoliation during winter to prevent further dryness and irritation.

Use a gentle exfoliator once a week to remove dead skin cells and promote cell turnover.

Choose exfoliators with moisturizing properties to enhance hydration.

- HYDRATION FROM WITHIN:

Stay hydrated by drinking an adequate amount of water throughout the day.

Consume foods rich in water content, such as fruits and vegetables, to support overall skin

hydration.

Herbal teas and warm water with lemon can also contribute to internal hydration.

- SPECIALIZED SKINCARE PRODUCTS:

Consider incorporating specialized skincare products, such as hydrating serums and masks,
into your routine.

Use overnight masks for intense hydration while you sleep.

Look for products with ingredients like ceramides, which help strengthen the skin's natural

barrier.

- AVOIDING HARSH INGREDIENTS:

Choose skincare products free from harsh ingredients, such as alcohol and fragrances, which

can exacerbate winter skin issues.

Opt for products labeled "fragrance-free" or "hypoallergenic" to minimize the risk of irritation.

Conduct patch tests when introducing new products to ensure compatibility with your skin.

Nurturing your skin during the winter season requires a thoughtful and consistent skincare

routine. By incorporating hydrating products, protecting your skin from harsh weather, and

maintaining a balance of moisture, you can ensure that your skin stays healthy, radiant, and resilient throughout the colder months. Embrace these winter skincare tips to keep your skin

glowing even in the face of chilly temperatures.

CHAPTER FOUR : BALANCING NUTRITION

As winter blankets the world in snow and brings a chill to the air, the importance of nutrition

takes center stage in maintaining health and vitality. The colder months often come with a

natural inclination towards comforting, hearty meals, but it's crucial to strike a balance that

nourishes the body and supports overall well-being. In this guide, we'll explore the art of

balancing nutrition during winter, ensuring that you not only stay warm but thrive in the midst of

the frosty season.

- EMBRACE SEASONAL PRODUCE:

Winter brings a bounty of seasonal fruits and vegetables rich in essential nutrients.

Incorporate winter superfoods like kale, Brussels sprouts, citrus fruits, and sweet potatoes into

your meals.

Experiment with hearty winter squash and root vegetables to add variety and nutritional value to your diet.

- **HYDRATE WITH WARM BEVERAGES:**

Combat winter dryness by staying hydrated with warm beverages.

Enjoy herbal teas, warm water with lemon, and nourishing broths to keep your body hydrated.

Limit the intake of caffeinated and sugary drinks that can contribute to dehydration.

- **BALANCED MACRONUTRIENTS:**

Ensure a balance of macronutrients in your meals, including carbohydrates, proteins, and

healthy fats.

Choose complex carbohydrates like whole grains, quinoa, and oats for sustained energy.

Include lean proteins such as poultry, fish, legumes, and nuts to support muscle health.

- **VITAMIN D-RICH FOODS:**

With reduced sunlight exposure, incorporate foods rich in vitamin D into your diet.

Include fatty fish like salmon and mackerel, fortified dairy products, and egg yolks to maintain optimal vitamin D levels.

Consider vitamin D supplements, especially if your exposure to natural sunlight is limited.

- IMMUNE-BOOSTING NUTRIENTS:

Strengthen your immune system with foods rich in vitamins C and E, zinc, and antioxidants.

Include citrus fruits, berries, nuts, seeds, and leafy greens to provide a nutritional shield against

winter illnesses.

Experiment with warming spices like ginger and turmeric, known for their immune-boosting

properties.

- MINDFUL EATING PRACTICES:

Practice mindful eating by savoring each bite and paying attention to hunger and fullness cues.

Avoid overindulging in comfort foods by cultivating a balanced approach to meals.

Enjoy meals in a calm and relaxed environment, fostering a positive relationship with food.

- COMFORTING AND NUTRIENT-RICH SOUPS:

Warm up with nutrient-dense soups that combine seasonal vegetables, lean proteins, and whole

grains.

Experiment with different soup recipes to ensure a variety of flavors and nutritional benefits.

Homemade soups provide not only warmth but also an opportunity to control ingredients for

optimal nutrition.

- LIMIT PROCESSED AND SUGARY FOODS:

Minimize the intake of processed and sugary foods that can contribute to inflammation and

energy crashes.

Opt for natural sweeteners like honey or maple syrup in moderation.

Read labels carefully and choose whole, minimally processed foods whenever possible.

Balancing nutrition during the winter is about more than just staying warm; it's about nourishing

your body to thrive in the cold. By embracing seasonal produce, staying hydrated with warm

beverages, and incorporating a variety of nutrient-rich foods, you can ensure that your winter meals are both comforting and health-supportive. Let this guide be your companion in creating a

winter nutrition plan that not only sustains you through the chill but also contributes to your

overall well-being.

CHAPTER FIVE : MINDFUL MENTAL HEALTH

As winter wraps the world in its icy embrace, the importance of mindful mental health practices

becomes paramount. The colder months, often associated with shorter days and longer nights,

can impact our mood and well-being. In this guide, we'll explore the art of cultivating mindful

mental health during winter – a journey that goes beyond simply surviving the chill, but actively

thriving in the midst of the season's unique challenges.

- EMBRACE THE WINTER MINDFULLY:

Approach winter with an open and mindful mindset, acknowledging its unique offerings and

challenges.

Cultivate a positive attitude by focusing on the beauty of winter landscapes, the warmth of cozy

moments, and the joy of seasonal activities.

- **NATURAL LIGHT EXPOSURE:**

Combat the winter blues by maximizing exposure to natural light during the day.

Spend time outdoors, even if it's a brief walk, to benefit from sunlight, which plays a crucial role

in regulating mood and circadian rhythms.

Consider light therapy lamps to supplement natural light exposure, especially on darker days.

- **MINDFUL BREATHING EXERCISES:**

Practice mindful breathing exercises to reduce stress and promote relaxation.

Incorporate deep belly breathing, box breathing, or guided mindfulness meditations into your

daily routine.

These exercises can be done indoors, providing a quick and effective way to center yourself

amidst winter's hustle.

- **CONNECT WITH NATURE:**

Engage with nature mindfully, whether it's observing snowfall, listening to the crunch of snow underfoot, or simply appreciating the stillness of a winter landscape.

Nature connection has been linked to improved mental well-being, so embrace winter as an

opportunity for mindful communion with the natural world.

- WINTER SELF-CARE RITUALS:

Develop winter-specific self-care rituals that cater to the needs of the season.

Enjoy a warm bath with soothing essential oils, indulge in a cozy reading nook, or practice

gentle yoga by the fireplace.

Identify activities that bring comfort and relaxation during the colder months.

- SOCIAL CONNECTION:

Combat feelings of isolation by maintaining social connections, even if it's through virtual

means.

Schedule regular video calls, participate in online communities, or organize virtual game nights

with friends and family.

Social interaction contributes significantly to mental well-being, especially during periods of

reduced outdoor activity.

- MINDFUL EATING PRACTICES:

Practice mindful eating by savoring each bite, paying attention to flavors, and eating without distraction.

Choose nutrient-dense foods that support both physical and mental health.

Be aware of emotional eating triggers and cultivate a mindful approach to nourishing your body.

- SET REALISTIC GOALS:

Set achievable goals for the winter season, whether they are related to personal growth, hobbies, or wellness.

Break larger goals into smaller, manageable tasks to maintain a sense of accomplishment.

Mindfully celebrate achievements and progress, no matter how small.

Cultivating mindful mental health during winter is about embracing the season with intentionality, resilience, and self-compassion. By incorporating mindfulness practices, connecting with nature,

and prioritizing self-care rituals, you can navigate the colder months with a sense of calm and

purpose. Let this guide be your companion on the journey to mindful well-being, helping you not

only endure the winter but truly thrive in its unique embrace.

CHAPTER SIX : HEALTHY SLEEP HABIT

As winter blankets the world in a snowy embrace, the importance of healthy sleep habits

becomes even more pronounced. The colder months invite us to indulge in cozy blankets and

longer nights, but maintaining a consistent and restful sleep routine is crucial for overall

well-being. In this guide, we'll delve into the art of nurturing healthy sleep habits during winter,

ensuring that you not only stay warm but wake up revitalized and ready to embrace the day.

CONSISTENT SLEEP SCHEDULE:
- Establish a consistent sleep schedule, going to bed and waking up at the same time each day.

- Align your sleep routine with natural light exposure to regulate your body's internal clock.
- Consistency reinforces your circadian rhythm, promoting better sleep quality.

CREATE A COZY SLEEP ENVIRONMENT:
- Design a sleep-friendly environment by keeping your bedroom dark, quiet, and cool.
- Invest in cozy, winter-appropriate bedding to enhance comfort and warmth.
- Consider blackout curtains to minimize external light and create an ideal sleep sanctuary.

LIMIT SCREEN TIME BEFORE BED:
- Reduce exposure to screens at least an hour before bedtime.
- The blue light emitted from electronic devices can interfere with melatonin production, making it harder to fall asleep.
- Instead, engage in relaxing activities such as reading a book or practicing gentle stretches.

WARM-UP YOUR SLEEP ROUTINE:
- Incorporate calming rituals into your evening routine to signal to your body that it's time to wind down.
- Enjoy a warm bath, practice relaxation exercises, or sip on a caffeine-free herbal tea to promote relaxation.
- Creating a soothing pre-sleep routine can signal to your body that it's time for rest.

MINDFUL BREATHING FOR SLEEP:

- Practice mindful breathing exercises or guided meditations to calm the mind and relax the body.
- Focusing on deep, rhythmic breaths can alleviate stress and prepare your body for a restful night's sleep.
- Consider integrating mindfulness practices into your bedtime routine.

LIMIT STIMULANTS AND HEAVY MEALS:
- Avoid consuming stimulants such as caffeine and nicotine close to bedtime.
- Opt for a light snack if hungry, avoiding heavy meals that can disrupt sleep.
- Moderating food and beverage intake before bedtime contributes to a more comfortable and uninterrupted sleep.

EXERCISE REGULARLY:
- Engage in regular physical activity, but aim to complete your workout at least a few hours before bedtime.
- Exercise promotes better sleep quality and can help regulate sleep-wake cycles.
- Gentle activities like yoga or a calming evening walk can be particularly beneficial.

CREATE A SLEEP-INDUCING ATMOSPHERE:
- Utilize calming scents, such as lavender or chamomile, through essential oils, diffusers, or scented candles.
- Experiment with white noise machines or calming nature sounds to drown out disruptive noises.
- Tailor your sleep environment to promote relaxation and a sense of tranquility.

Nurturing healthy sleep habits during winter is a cornerstone of overall well-being. By establishing a consistent sleep schedule, creating a cozy sleep environment, and incorporating relaxation techniques into your bedtime routine, you can enhance the quality of your sleep and wake up feeling refreshed, even on the coldest winter mornings. Let this guide be your companion in fostering healthy sleep habits, ensuring that you not only endure the winter nights but embrace them with restful serenity.

CHAPTER SEVEN : WINTER HYDRATION

While winter is often associated with chilly temperatures and snow-covered landscapes, it's essential to recognize that hydration remains a crucial aspect of overall well-being during this season. The colder weather, combined with indoor heating, can lead to dehydration, affecting various aspects of health. In this guide, we'll explore the art of winter hydration, ensuring that you stay adequately nourished and thrive in the face of the frosty season.

Cold Weather and Dehydration:
- Cold weather can mask the body's signals of thirst, leading to reduced water intake.
- Indoor heating systems contribute to dry air, increasing the risk of dehydration.
- Despite the colder temperatures, it's crucial to maintain hydration levels to support various bodily functions.

Drink Warm Beverages:
- Embrace warm beverages to stay hydrated while also enjoying the comforting aspect of winter drinks.

- Herbal teas, warm water with lemon, and broths not only provide hydration but also contribute to overall well-being.
- Limit excessive consumption of caffeinated and sugary beverages, as they can contribute to dehydration.

Hydrate from Within:
- Consume water-rich foods to supplement your hydration, including fruits like watermelon, oranges, and berries.
- Incorporate hydrating vegetables like cucumber and celery into your meals.
- Soups and stews with a high water content can also contribute to your overall fluid intake.

Stay Consistently Hydrated:
- Establish a consistent hydration routine by drinking water throughout the day.
- Carry a reusable water bottle to encourage regular sipping, even if you're not feeling thirsty.
- Set reminders to drink water, especially if you're engaged in indoor activities that may distract you from staying hydrated.

Limit Dehydrating Substances:
- Be mindful of substances that can contribute to dehydration, such as excessive caffeine and alcohol.
- Moderation is key when consuming beverages that have diuretic effects, as they can increase fluid loss.

Humidifier Use:

- Integrate humidifiers into your indoor environment to combat the dry air caused by heating systems.
- Optimal indoor humidity levels contribute to both respiratory health and skin hydration.
- Place humidifiers in frequently used areas, such as bedrooms and living rooms, for consistent hydration.

Monitor Hydration Levels:

- Pay attention to signs of dehydration, including dark urine, dry skin, and a feeling of thirst.
- If engaging in outdoor winter activities, be mindful of increased fluid needs due to physical exertion.
- Adjust your fluid intake based on your activity level and individual hydration requirements.

Incorporate Electrolytes:

- If engaging in winter sports or activities that involve sweating, consider incorporating electrolyte-rich beverages.
- Electrolytes help maintain the body's fluid balance and are particularly important during physical exertion in cold weather.

Winter hydration is a fundamental component of maintaining overall health and well-being during the colder months. By adopting mindful hydration practices, drinking warm beverages, and staying consistently hydrated, you can ensure that your body remains nourished and resilient in the face of winter's unique challenges. Let this guide be your companion in embracing winter hydration, supporting your body, and thriving in the cold.

CHAPTER EIGHT : SEASONAL ILLNESS

As winter descends with its icy winds and frosty

landscapes, the risk of seasonal illnesses

looms large. Cold and flu viruses thrive in colder

temperatures, and the confined indoor spaces

during winter, it provides an environment conducive to the

spread of infections. In this guide,

we'll explore strategies to fortify your defenses against

seasonal illnesses, ensuring that you not

only endure the cold months but emerge resilient and

healthy.

- HAND HYGIENE AND RESPIRATORY
  ETIQUETTE:

Practice rigorous hand hygiene by washing hands

frequently with soap and water for at least 20

seconds.

Use hand sanitizers containing at least 60% alcohol when soap and water are unavailable.

Follow proper respiratory etiquette by covering your mouth

and nose with a tissue or your elbow

when coughing or sneezing.

- GET VACCINATED:

Consider getting vaccinated against the flu to protect

yourself and others from influenza.

Stay updated on recommended vaccinations, including

those for pneumonia and other

preventable diseases.

Consult with healthcare professionals to determine the

appropriate vaccines for your specific

health needs.

- BOOST IMMUNITY WITH NUTRITION:

Support your immune system with a nutrient-rich diet

containing vitamins C and E, zinc, and

antioxidants.

Incorporate fruits, vegetables, nuts, and seeds into your

meals to provide essential nutrients.

Consider dietary supplements, especially vitamin D, to

address potential deficiencies during the

winter months.

- STAY ACTIVE FOR IMMUNE HEALTH:

Engage in regular physical activity to boost immune

function and overall health.

Moderate exercise has been shown to enhance the

immune response and reduce the risk of

respiratory infections.

Choose winter-friendly activities like indoor workouts, yoga,

or brisk walks to stay active.

- ADEQUATE SLEEP FOR RECOVERY:

Prioritize sufficient and quality sleep to support your body's

recovery and immune function.

Maintain a consistent sleep schedule and create a

comfortable sleep environment conducive to

restful sleep.

Lack of sleep can compromise the immune system,

making you more susceptible to illnesses.

- MANAGE STRESS TO REDUCE
  SUSCEPTIBILITY:

Practice stress management techniques such as

mindfulness, meditation, or deep breathing

exercises.

Chronic stress can weaken the immune response, so

prioritizing mental well-being is crucial

during the winter months.

Find activities that bring relaxation and joy to counteract

the stresses of the season.

- PROPER HYDRATION FOR IMMUNE SUPPORT:

Stay adequately hydrated to support your immune system

and maintain overall health.

Drink water, herbal teas, and broths to stay hydrated,

especially in heated indoor environments.

Adequate hydration helps the body flush out toxins and

supports the proper functioning of

immune cells.

- LIMIT EXPOSURE TO SICK INDIVIDUALS:

Minimize close contact with individuals showing symptoms

of illness.

Practice social distancing and wear masks in crowded or

enclosed spaces to reduce the risk of

viral transmission.

Stay informed about local health guidelines and adhere to

recommended precautions.

Defending against seasonal illnesses in winter requires a

multifaceted approach that combines

hygiene practices, vaccination, immune-boosting nutrition,

and lifestyle habits that support

overall well-being. By adopting these strategies, you can

fortify your defenses, reduce the risk of

infections, and navigate the winter season with resilience

and health. Let this guide be your

resource in creating a winter wellness plan that prioritizes

your immune health and ensures a

healthy and thriving season.

CONCLUSION

As winter blankets the world in frosty landscapes,

Maintaining good health becomes paramount.

Embracing a holistic approach to well-being during the

winter months involves a combination of

practices. Regular exercise, balanced nutrition, and

adequate hydration contribute to a robust

immune system, helping ward off seasonal illnesses.

Adequate rest and sleep are equally

crucial, allowing the body to rejuvenate and strengthen its

defenses. Additionally, practicing

good hygiene, such as frequent handwashing, further

safeguards against winter viruses. By

adopting these habits, one can navigate the winter season

with resilience, ensuring a healthier

and a more enjoyable experience amidst the chilly

temperatures.
Moreover, incorporating immune-boosting foods into your

diet, rich in vitamins and antioxidants,

provides an extra layer of protection against common

winter ailments. Warm beverages like

herbal teas and soups not only keep you cozy but also

contribute to hydration and overall

well-being. Don't underestimate the importance of

maintaining mental health during the

winter—engage in activities that bring joy, connect with

loved ones, and consider spending time

outdoors when weather permits.

It's also advisable to stay informed about seasonal health

precautions, such as getting flu

vaccinations and keeping an eye on local health

advisories. Embracing a positive mindset and

adapting healthy habits can turn the winter season into an

opportunity for self-care and personal

growth. Remember, a well-nourished body and a positive

mindset work hand in hand to create a

resilient and thriving state of health throughout the winter

months. By prioritizing your well-being,

you can not only survive but truly thrive in the winter

season.

In addition, safeguarding against the winter blues involves

acknowledging the impact of reduced

sunlight on mood and energy levels. Consider spending

time outdoors during daylight hours,

even if it's just for a short walk, to benefit from natural light

exposure. Incorporating vitamin D

supplements, as recommended by healthcare

professionals, can also help mitigate the effects

of decreased sunlight.

Furthermore, staying vigilant about respiratory health is

crucial in the winter, as cold and dry air

can exacerbate respiratory issues. Hydrate your

respiratory system by using a humidifier,

especially while sleeping, to maintain optimal moisture

levels in the air. Practicing good

respiratory hygiene, such as covering your mouth and

nose when coughing or sneezing, further

contributes to a healthier winter environment.

In conclusion, by embracing a comprehensive approach

that encompasses physical, mental,

and respiratory well-being, you can fortify your health

during the winter months. These proactive

measures not only shield you from seasonal challenges

but also empower you to enjoy the

beauty and uniqueness of winter with vitality and

resilience.